Easy Exercises

Simple Workout Routine For Busy People In The Office, At Home, Or On The Road

Patrick Barrett

Copyright © 2012 Patrick Barrett

All rights reserved.

ISBN-10: 1478200278
ISBN-13: 978-1478200277

CONTENTS

Introduction	1
What Can Exercise Do For You?	4
What Are We Going To Do About it?	10
One More Quick Note Before The Good Stuff	12
I Lied! One Last Thing	14
Part 1: Jumping Jacks	17
Part 2: Trunk Twists	19
Part 3: Toe Touch Squats	22
Part 3 Alternate: Deadlift Press Squats	30
Part 4: Pushups/Plank (Optional)	38
Part 5: Curl Press (Optional)	42
Sets, Reps, and Schedule	45
Rest	50
Challenge Yourself	54
Don't Undervalue This	57
Easy Exercise As A Supplement	60

Basic Diet	62
General Tips	66
Conclusion	68
About The Author	69
Other Books By Patrick Barrett	70

> "Those who think they have not time for bodily exercise will sooner or later have to find time for illness."
>
> *-Edward Stanley*

Books by Patrick Barrett:

Natural Exercise: Basic Bodyweight Training and Calisthenics for Strength and Weight-Loss

The Natural Diet: Simple Nutritional Advice For Optimal Health In The Modern World

How To Do A Handstand: From the Basic Exercises To The Free Standing Handstand Pushup

Best Ab Exercises: Abdominal Workout Routine For Core Strength And A Flat Stomach

Hand And Forearm Exercises: Grip Strength Workout And Training Routine

Advanced Bodyweight Exercises: An Intense Full Body Workout In A Home Or Gym

One Arm Pull Up: Bodyweight Training And Exercise Program For One Arm Pull Ups And Chin Ups

Easy Exercises: Simple Workout Routine For Busy People In The Office, At Home, Or On The Road

Disclaimer:

This book was not written or reviewed by a doctor, personal trainer, dietitian, or other licensed person. Always consult with your doctor before beginning any exercise routine or implementing any change in your diet or medication.

INTRODUCTION

Hi, I'm Patrick Barrett, and I'd like to thank you for buying this book.

Finding an exercise routine to stick to—and then sticking to it—is truly one of the best decisions you can make for yourself. If you want to be healthy, regular exercise is an absolute must.

In this book, you're going to learn everything you need to know to make full-body exercise a regular part of your life —even if you've never exercised before, even if you don't have much time, and even if you're not trying to become Arnold Schwarzenegger.

Though a lot of emphasis today is put on developing a "beach body" or looking like a movie star—and getting there as quickly as possible, no matter the cost—there is also a huge health benefit for people who do any kind of regular exercise, even if that exercise does not result in rapid, dramatic changes in your physical appearance.

In fact, exercise programs that are too extreme can have detrimental effects down the road for many people.

The purpose of this book is just to teach you a simple, short, convenient full-body exercise routine, and to get you exercising regularly. It doesn't take much time, and it can be done with little or no equipment. It might be a jumping-off point from which you start getting much more into exercise, or if working out is less of an interest for you and you want to keep it simple, it might be the only routine you do for the rest of your life.

Once you're on board and you can execute that routine, the choice is yours. You can continue with the simple routine indefinitely and enjoy the many health benefits of regular exercise (which we'll cover in the next chapter), or if you like you can try any of a number of different, more challenging variations, which we'll discuss later in the book.

If you choose to stick with the simple routine, your body will thank you—improved circulation will keep your blood and your body cleaner, and more frequent use will make your muscles and joints stronger and healthier. If you stick with it and eat right, you will even notice a real difference in your physique over time.

If you choose to increase the level of difficulty with some of the progressions from later on in the book, you'll enjoy those same benefits with even greater improvements in strength and physical appearance.

Either way, you'll learn a useful, long-term routine that delivers useful, long-term results.

Now let's get started.

Other Books by Patrick Barrett:

Natural Exercise: *Basic Bodyweight Training and Calisthenics for Strength and Weight-Loss*

The Natural Diet: *Simple Nutritional Advice For Optimal Health In The Modern World*

How To Do A Handstand: *From the Basic Exercises To The Free Standing Handstand Pushup*

One Arm Pull Up: *Bodyweight Training And Exercise Program For One Arm Pull Ups And Chin Ups*

Advanced Bodyweight Exercises: *An Intense Full Body Workout In A Home Or Gym*

Best Ab Exercises: *Abdominal Workout Routine For Core Strength And A Flat Stomach*

Hand And Forearm Exercises: *Grip Strength Workout And Training Routine*

WHAT CAN EXERCISE DO FOR YOU?

There are so many people who would love to find a simple exercise routine that they can stick to.

That should come as no surprise, really, because there's a ton of money being spent to convince people they should be exercising. You can't open a magazine or turn on a television without being bombarded with ads for new workout routines or equipment that are supposed to transform your life.

One of the big problems that arises from this hyper-marketing is that the general public (that's you and me) develops a distorted understanding of what really is so important about exercise—and how much exercise it takes to start to experience some of those important benefits.

If you watch one of those infomercials, or you read one of those ads, you come away thinking that exercise will accomplish two things for you: (1) it will develop your muscles so that they become larger and/or more toned, and (2) it will cause you to burn off excess fat.

Of course, both of these are possible, but there is a lot more going on here.

Then, the ad will tend to propose one of two approaches: the really easy routine that works out one part of your body but doesn't actually produce reliable results (see almost every butt or ab workout gadget ever made), or the routine that does produce results, but is very strenuous and involved.

People who follow either of these often quit from frustration; either they take the easy route and quit because nothing happens, or they take the hard route and quit because it's just too difficult and time-consuming.

The result is that many people who could be benefitting from a simpler, shorter, full-body exercise routine are instead doing the worst thing—nothing—because they think it's too difficult to do an amount of exercise that's actually worthwhile.

So let's discuss some of the less-known benefits of exercise, so that we can then have a better appreciation for the importance of a regular workout routine—not as a difficult luxury whose only purpose is to create a more attractive body, but as an absolute necessity which is less demanding than you might imagine, and which will increase your overall health and quality of life.

To understand the importance of exercise, first we need to understand the importance of circulation. You probably know that the term "circulation" describes the way blood travels through your body. Did you also know that it is this circulating action which allows your blood—and therefore your body—to be cleaned?

Let's take a step back to make sure we get a thorough understanding of how all this works. I feel like I should note that the human body is incredibly complex and some of these processes are a little simplified here, but not in a way that makes any difference to this discussion.

We'll start with the cell. Of course, your body is made up of all different kinds of cells that all have different jobs to do. When they do those jobs, they produce waste products. These toxins need to be cleared away so that your cells—and the organs that are made up of those cells—can continue to do their work effectively.

When your blood comes circulating around your body, it does many important things, but we'll focus on two. One, it brings fresh oxygen and nutrients, so that your cells can continue to function properly, and two, it also clears away the waste products, so they don't build up and make you sick.

So, your blood continues to travel its way around your body, dropping off oxygen and nutrients, and picking up waste. When it gets to the kidneys, the blood is cleaned out—your kidneys clean all that waste from your blood, and soon your body gets rid of it as urine. Then your blood is clean, and it can make another trip around you body, delivering nutrients and gathering more waste to be again cleaned out and eliminated.

This process is absolutely crucial. In fact, if your body becomes unable to clean away these waste products, you will get sick and die. However, even if it's not severe enough to kill you or make you outright sick, it can have a negative effect on your overall health; you might have low energy levels, or you might get sick easily, you might even be forgetful or depressed .

You've probably heard here and there that exercise can help to alleviate any or all of these problems.

Think of it this way: imagine that you have five garbage cans around your house, and you don't get around to cleaning them that often. Imagine that as the days go by, these garbage cans get fuller and fuller with trash—banana peels, egg shells, chicken bones, who knows what else.

Because you don't make your way around the house to empty those cans, they overflow and get disgusting—there's bugs and odor and bacteria all over, which starts to make life less pleasant in your home.

Now let's imagine that you have those same garbage cans, but you make a trip around the house each day to empty them. Because they are frequently emptied, they never get close to full, and you never have any trouble with insects or bad smells or anything like that.

Well, that's how it goes in your body, too. The more often your blood circulates through your body, the more often your blood picks up waste, and then gets cleaned out. The cleaner your blood is, the more of your cells' waste products it can carry away on each trip. That means your cells, your organs, and your blood are cleaner, which means that your body can do all the things it needs to do, better.

Better circulation can lead to higher energy levels, better moods, a sharper mind, a stronger immune system, better sleep—all kinds of things—because your blood and organs are not, metaphorically speaking, knee-deep in their own garbage.

So now we see one of the hugely important health benefits of exercise that has little to do with burning fat or building muscle: improved circulation and a cleaner body. Sure, those things will help you burn fat and build muscle too, but there's much more to it than that.

Another benefit of exercise is that it causes you to breathe deeper. Deeper breathing helps to promote better circulation (which we now know is important) and it can also provide more oxygen to your blood, and therefore to your cells, which can further promote your cellular (and therefore overall) health.

Also, the simple act of using your muscles and joints, even for light exercise, allows them to get stronger and healthier, and also to stay stronger and healthier for longer.

When you do an exercise routine that uses your whole body, your circulation increases much more than it would if you were just exercising one particular part (like your abs or your butt, for example).

The upshot of all of this is that even a light workout routine that uses your whole body (and that you actually stick to) can provide great benefits to you even if it's not quite strenuous enough to create a dramatic change in your appearance—although it can change that too, it just takes some time!

There is another important aspect to consider here. In the modern world, the majority of people have to do very little physical labor to get by.

Easy Exercises

Centuries ago, simply staying alive required very hard work. There was much more walking, most jobs required a lot more physical labor, and even leisure activities required you to get up and move around. Simply put, you didn't have a choice when it came to being physically active.

Today, though, many people spend their work and leisure time on a phone or sitting down in front of a screen. We get around in cars and buses. Because of advances in technology, we now have the choice—a very popular choice—to do almost no physical labor in our daily lives.

That means your blood gets around much less, which means waste builds up in your body, which means your body is unable to function at anywhere near an optimal level. Add that to the fact that poor diet frequently goes hand in hand with a sedentary lifestyle, which means that in addition to being stuck in their own waste, your cells are getting low quality nutrients, and it's no wonder that so many people are—to put it bluntly—fat, sick, tired, and depressed.

It also means that actively making the decision to exercise regularly is more important now than it has ever been—because if you don't make that decision, modern conveniences will allow you to do less physical work than ever before, which is terrible for your whole body!

This is not about losing weight and toning up. It's about your quality of life.

So what are we going to do about all of this? Now that you know what's on the line, why is this workout different from any other?

That sounds like a great topic for the next chapter.

WHAT ARE WE GOING TO DO ABOUT IT?

So now we've established that there is a crucial benefit to exercise which is completely separate from the desire to lose fat and build muscle, and that your body can start to experience this benefit even by doing light full-body exercise on a regular basis. What next?

Well, we are going to build a relatively quick, relatively simple exercise routine that you can do anywhere. Then you'll always be able to get in a full-body workout, which means you'll enjoy cleaner blood, cells, and organs, and a better quality of life.

One key component of this routine is that you will do just one set of each exercise. When people go to the gym, a lot of time is spent just waiting between sets so that their muscles can recover enough from the last set to do the next one. You'll be doing one set of each exercise, and moving right from one exercise to another, so you get the most out of the time you put in.

Over time, you will see weight loss and muscle development if you stick with it, and especially if you work in some of the more challenging stuff we talk about toward the end.

Along the way we'll discuss a lot of smaller, related topics so that you can get the most out of your new workout routine, and so that you'll be better equipped to make decisions about physical activity in the future.

ONE MORE QUICK NOTE BEFORE THE GOOD STUFF

Almost all of the workout routines I teach start out with a chapter on warming up and a chapter on stretching. Warming up and stretching are absolutely critical, especially for more intense workouts, to get the best possible results and also to keep from injuring yourself.

Warming up is basically light full-body exercise. It gets blood pumping through your muscles, and it limbers them up. Stretching is... well, stretching. It further prepares your muscles for the exercise, and helps you to avoid injury, especially when you're going to do strenuous exercise.

So, warming up and stretching are both important. They are also two things that make sticking to a good exercise routine difficult for many people, because they make your workout that much longer, and that much harder to fit into a busy schedule.

Easy Exercises

Well, this workout routine is, itself, relatively light exercise. So the warm up and the workout sort of go hand-in-hand, and you can't really tell where one ends and the other begins. To be clear, I'm not saying you don't need to warm up, but that the warm up is itself already part of the routine.

Also, stretching is less important here because it is light exercise. For example, you don't need to stretch out your muscles before you take a walk, do you? No, because walking is not strenuous. This is a little more strenuous than that, but there are also stretching motions built right in to the exercises you'll be doing, which will take care of your stretching needs for the sake of this routine.

So, through the magical convenience of this workout routine, the warm up, stretching, and exercise are all sort of combined into one. That way you still get everything you need, but you get it done in less time.

For that reason, I won't be singling out one portion of the routine as the "Warm Up," or one part as "Stretching," or anything like that, which is what I usually do in my books about more intense exercise; instead we'll just look at everything in sequence.

I just wanted to take a moment to explain that and let you know I've got you covered.

Now we've finally gotten to the good stuff—the actual routine!

I LIED! ONE LAST THING

To put it simply, the purpose of this book is to help busy people exercise regularly. It's a simple—but very important—goal, and its success can mean a huge difference in your health, well-being, and quality of life.

In order to achieve that goal, a busy person needs a routine which is challenging enough to be beneficial, but quick and convenient enough that it can be squeezed into any given day, no matter how packed that day already is.

One issue worth discussing briefly, though, is the potential variability in my audience. A busy person can be a 60-year-old lady who weighs 100 pounds and has never tried to exercise before in her life. It can also be a 220 pound, 23-year-old guy who can bench-press a semi-truck—and it can mean anything at all in between.

What I'm getting at here is that it can be difficult to present this material in a way that won't seem either way too hard, or way too easy, to at least one major chunk of my audience. So let me take the time right here to point out something you need to keep in mind:

This program can be beneficial for anybody.

Remember, the point here is to promote circulation and regular exercise, no matter who you are. If you are brand-new to exercise and some of this looks like it might be hard, don't worry—you can start out with numbers as low as you want (well, as long as you're still actually doing something) and then work your way up from there when you become able.

If you have a lot of experience, but not a lot of time, and you're looking for an efficient way to get in some daily exercise, you can increase the repetitions and/or use some of the more challenging variations we'll get into later to keep things interesting. Even if you need to add a hundred total repetitions to make it worth your while, at less than a couple of seconds per rep, it still only adds two or three minutes to the length of the workout, which should be very doable for anybody.

After all, you might be able to squat a house, but if you can no longer make time to get to the gym and actually do it, your strength and health will inevitably decline. This routine will keep you active every day, which might not give dramatic results in a few short weeks, but it will pay off huge in the long run.

Much of the writing here is probably aimed more at beginners than at those with a lot of workout experience. That's just because the beginners need a little more input. If you don't fit into that beginner category, rest assured that I've still got you covered.

The truest test of the value of this routine is just for you to do it. Read the book, and apply it to your daily life. Tweak the number of reps over the course of the first week or two, and once you hit the numerical sweet spot you'll have a simple routine that keeps you fit and active when your schedule just won't fit in anything else, whether you're new to exercise or not.

Now, let's actually take a look at this simple routine.

PART 1: JUMPING JACKS

Yup, we're going to start this off just like we're in gym class. Don't worry, it will get more interesting after this.

The fact of the matter is that jumping jacks are probably the best way to get your muscles warm without overtaxing them, especially if you aren't used to exercise. This exercise is used in the military, in organized sports, all over the place, and it's because it just works.

Almost everyone knows what a jumping jack is. All the same, let's take a look at some pictures so we know we're on the same page.

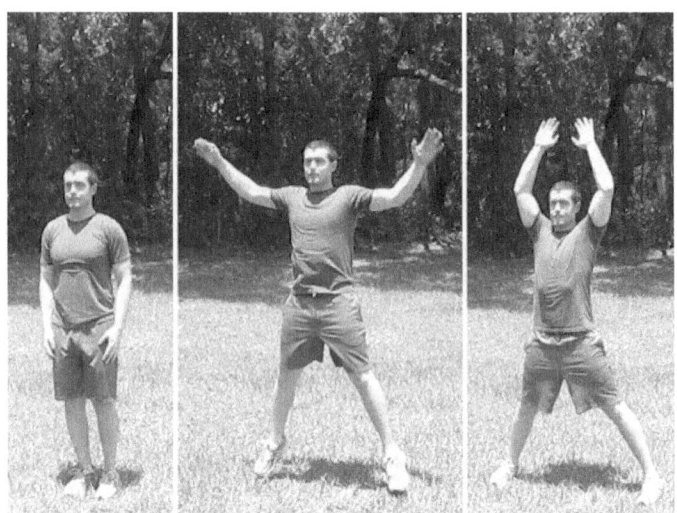

As you can see, you'll stand with your feet roughly shoulder-width apart, then jump up, while spreading your legs and lifting your arms straight above your head. Land with your feet spread and your arms up, and then do the movement in reverse, jumping back to the original position. That's one repetition.

You're going to do one set of these, and you want to do them until they just start to be a little taxing. That might be ten, it might be twenty, it might be 50 or more. Find that number, and do your one set, then move right to the next exercise.

PART 2: TRUNK TWISTS

Strength and flexibility in your abdomen and lower back are crucial. If you want to have good posture and avoid lower back pain, you must keep these muscles limber.

Trunk twists are great because they are a low-impact way to get all the muscles in your midsection working and stretching at the same time. Let's take a look at this movement.

Raise your arms straight out to your sides, and twist in a smooth, controlled motion to one side, and then to the other. Twisting to one side, to the other side, and back to the start is one repetition.

I can't stress enough that this movement needs to be slow and controlled, especially in the beginning. In this exercise, as with any exercise in this book or any other book I've written, always stay in control and only go as far you're comfortable going, especially in the beginning when you're getting used to it. You'll increase your range of motion with more practice, but there's no need to rush.

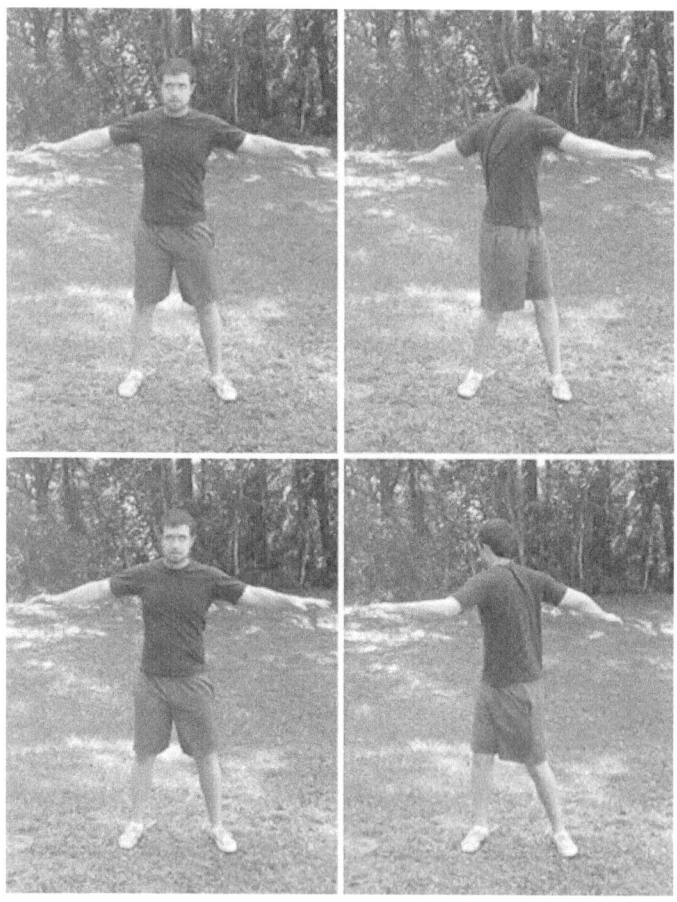

Your back, as you probably already know, is really important, and an uncontrolled twisting movement can cause you injury. There's no reason to be afraid of this, but especially if you're someone who isn't used to regular exercise, take this slow until you feel like you know what

Easy Exercises

you're doing. If you can only twist a little bit each way comfortably, that's fine. Just be patient and build up your range of motion over time.

After your jumping jacks, you want to do one set of these. Do enough that your midsection feels looser and more limber; probably around 10-25 will be good.

PART 3: TOE TOUCH SQUATS

These are the heart and soul of your simple workout. They are slightly more complex than the previous two exercises, so we'll spend a little more time looking at each part of the sequence.

Easy Exercises

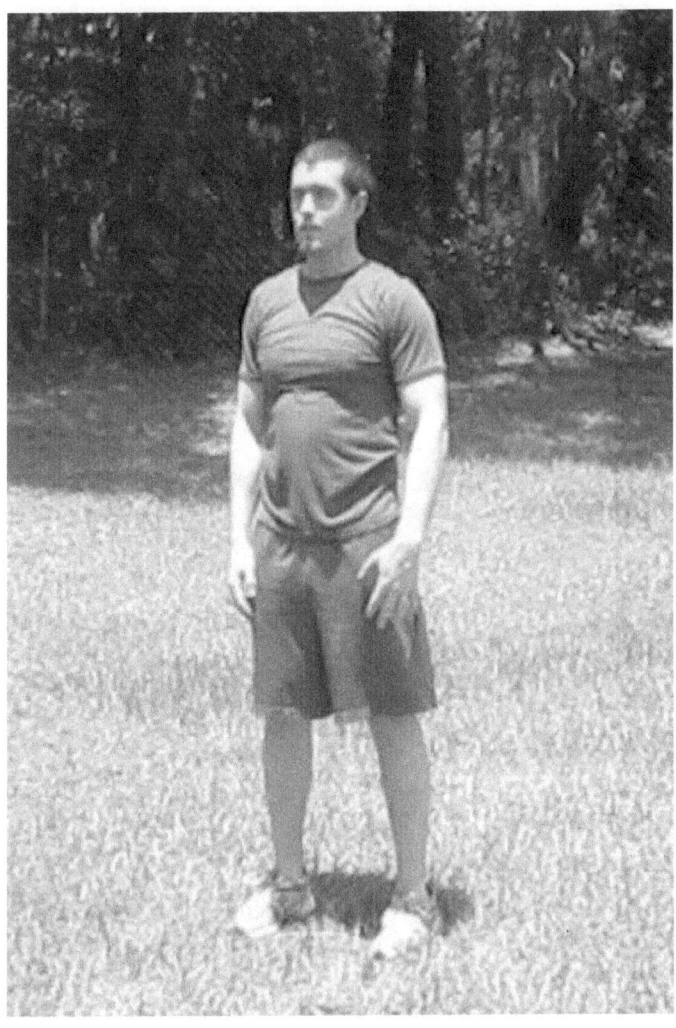

First, stand with your feet shoulder-width apart. Okay, so this first part is pretty easy.

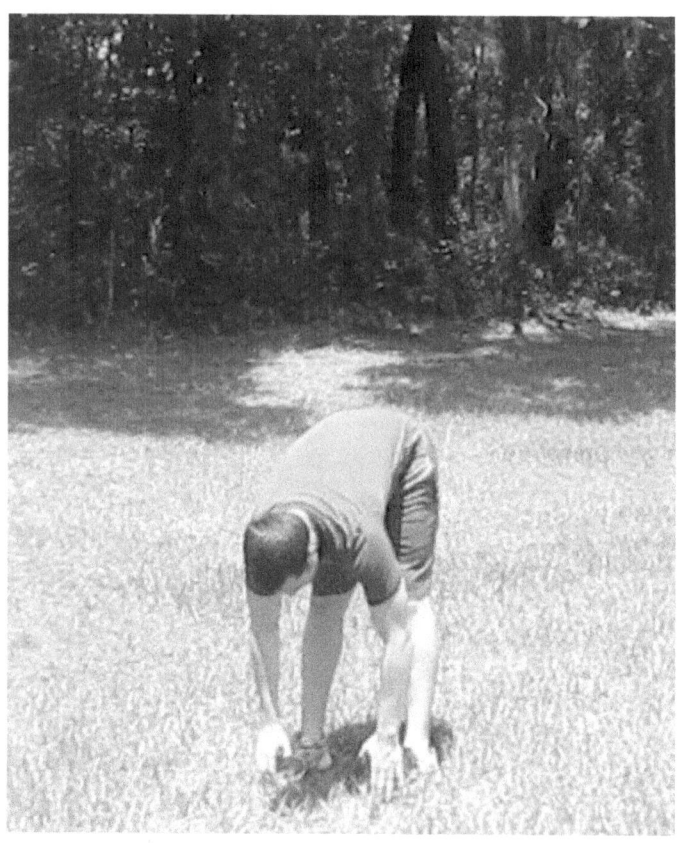

Then, keeping your legs straight, bend down at the waist and touch your toes. You may not actually be able to touch your toes (or, you may touch them easily). Just go down far enough that you start to feel a little stretch in your hamstrings, and, as always, go down gently and smoothly so you don't strain anything or pull a muscle.

Easy Exercises

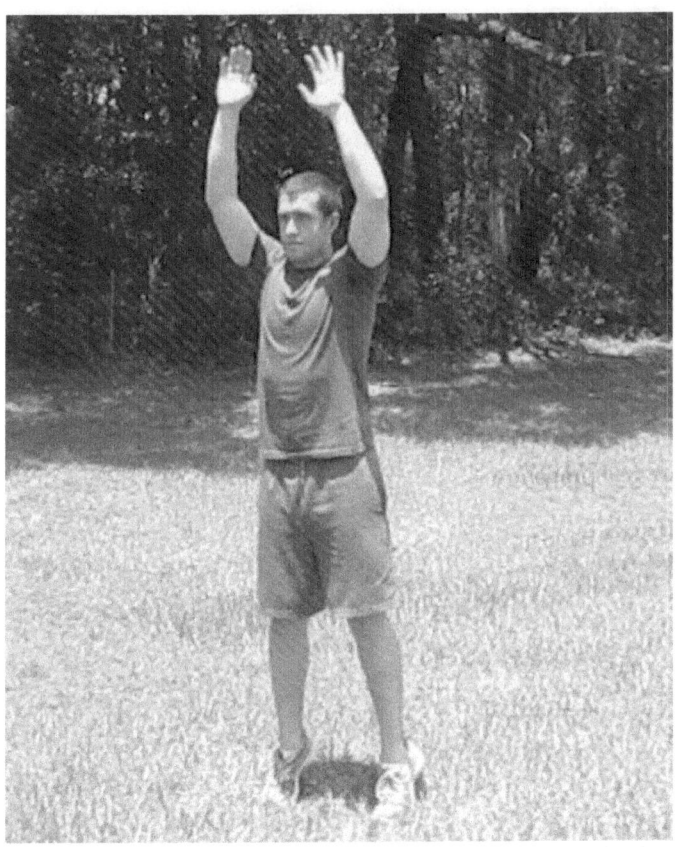

Continuing to keep your legs straight, stand back up and raise your hands above your head. Really stretch your hands and your whole body upward. Going up on your toes at this point is optional; it's not a bad thing to add but don't worry about it if it messes with your balance.

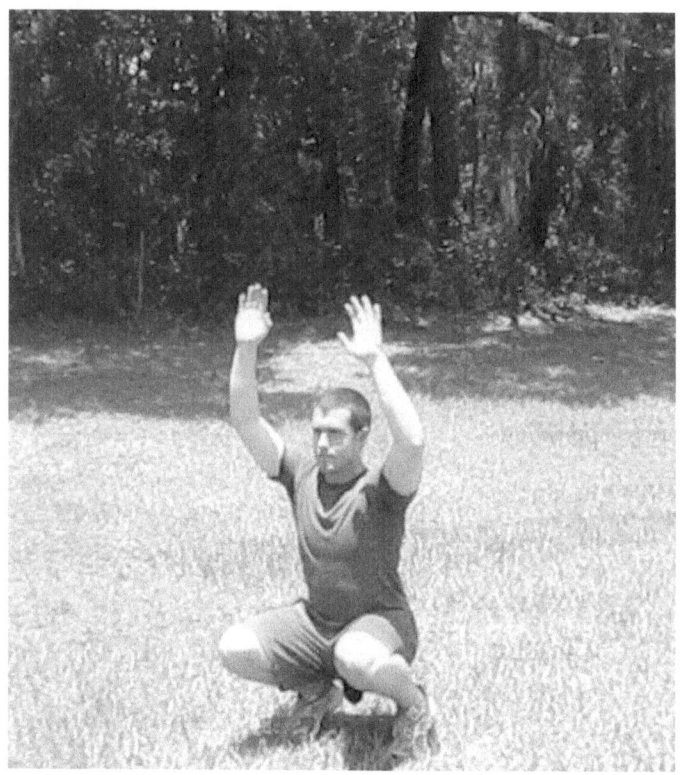

From there, squat all the way down as far as you can (hopefully until your butt is on your ankles, as pictured). If you can't go that far down, go down as far as you comfortably can, and try to increase your range of motion over time. It's okay if your heels come up as you squat down as low as you're comfortably able to.

Easy Exercises

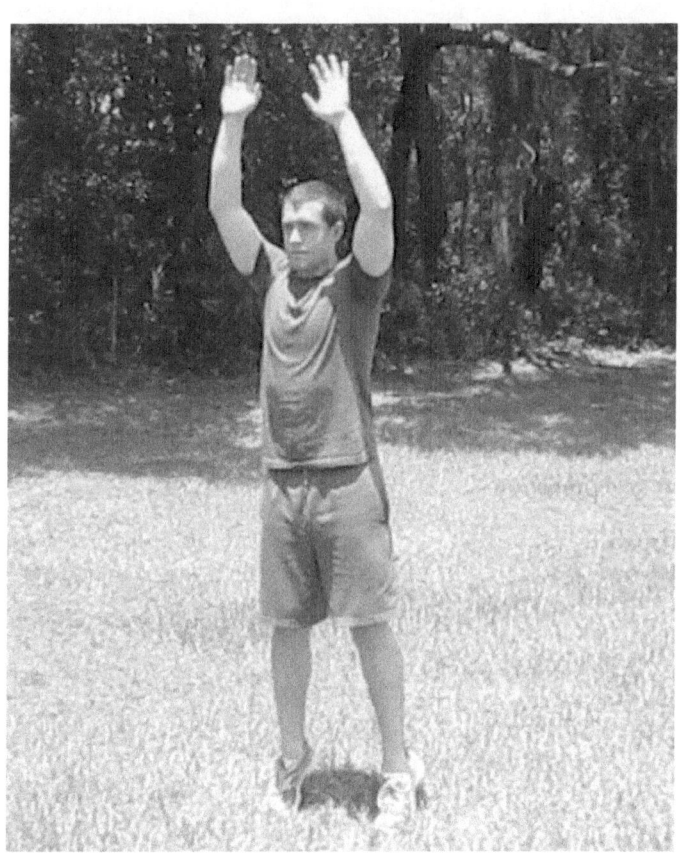

Keeping your arms above your head, stand back up. You've done one repetition.

Bend down and touch your toes again, and repeat.

Here's how it all looks together:

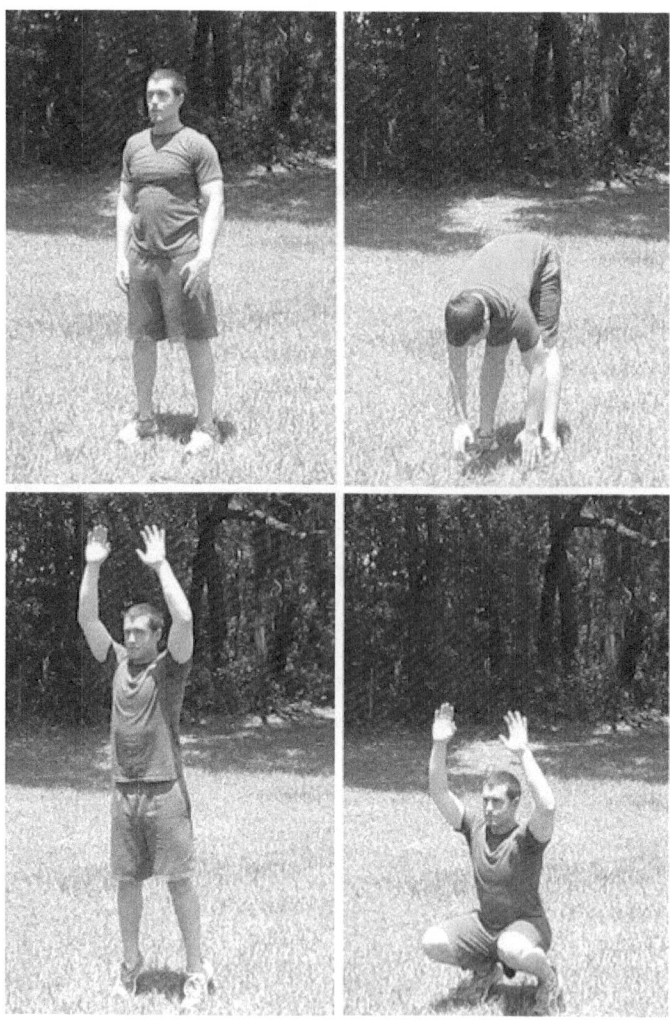

This is a surprisingly great exercise. A lower body workout is a great way to take advantage of the circulation-related benefits we discussed earlier, because the muscles in your legs are the largest in your body, so exercising them promotes circulation and deep breathing more than any other muscle group.

Furthermore, this exercise, by combining the toe touch and the squat, works out all the major muscle groups in your lower body at the same time—your butt, your hamstrings, and your quadriceps.

You will do one set of these until you start to feel a little bit fatigued. How many that takes will depend on your age, weight, and experience level with exercise, but it could be anywhere in the 5-25 range in the beginning. Be sure to increase that number after you've gotten used to the routine so it stays a little challenging.

Again, this is sort of the crux of this simple workout, so make sure you're pushing yourself a little bit.

PART 3 ALTERNATE: DEADLIFT PRESS SQUATS

In the last chapter, we talked about the core of the bodyweight version of this simple routine. In this chapter, we'll look at an alternative that uses weights.

Don't get me wrong—the point of this book is to teach you a convenient workout that you can do anywhere, and if you prefer to keep it simple and not get weights involved, you can certainly do that.

Having said that, some people will want a little variation, and in keeping with the theme of the book, this is a stripped-down, convenient version of weight-lifting, and you don't have to join a gym or even invest in a complete set of weights. A single pair of dumbbells (or a single barbell) that you can keep in your bedroom, your living room, or your office (or wherever is most convenient) will suffice.

Easy Exercises

This is similar to the routine in the previous chapter, just slightly adapted. So, instead of going through each step in the same detail, we'll just look at a series of pictures depicting the whole movement, and then I'll note any important points afterward:

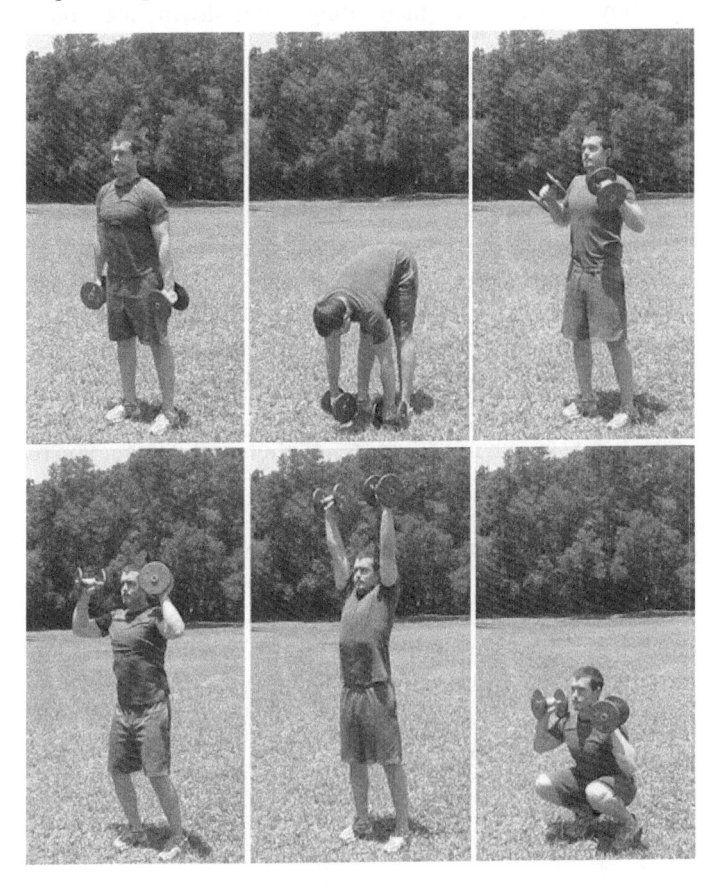

I've broken it down with a couple of extra pictures, but that's just to show you exactly where the weights are at each point in the exercise; this should be basically the same movement as the bodyweight version.

Once you get to the last picture in the sequence, follow the it back through in reverse—from the squat, stand and press the weight above your head, then lower the weight and bend down to touch your toes, then raise the weights back up above your head, then bring them down and squat again, and so on.

Be sure to use the same form we talked about in the last chapter. This shouldn't present any enormous challenge since you'll be using relatively light weights, but you always want to take it slow and easy in the beginning when you're getting used to a new movement, and that certainly applies here.

As you can see, you still go through the same basic toe touch and squat motion. The biggest difference is that the part where you lift your arms from your sides to up above your head is obviously more challenging, since you're holding weights.

In the picture, you can see that instead of keeping my hands raised above my head, as in the bodyweight routine, I have lowered the weights to my shoulders while squatting. If you are working with relatively light weight, or if you want more of a challenge, you can keep your arms raised above your head through the squatting motion, or you can keep them in the position shown above, like this:

Easy Exercises

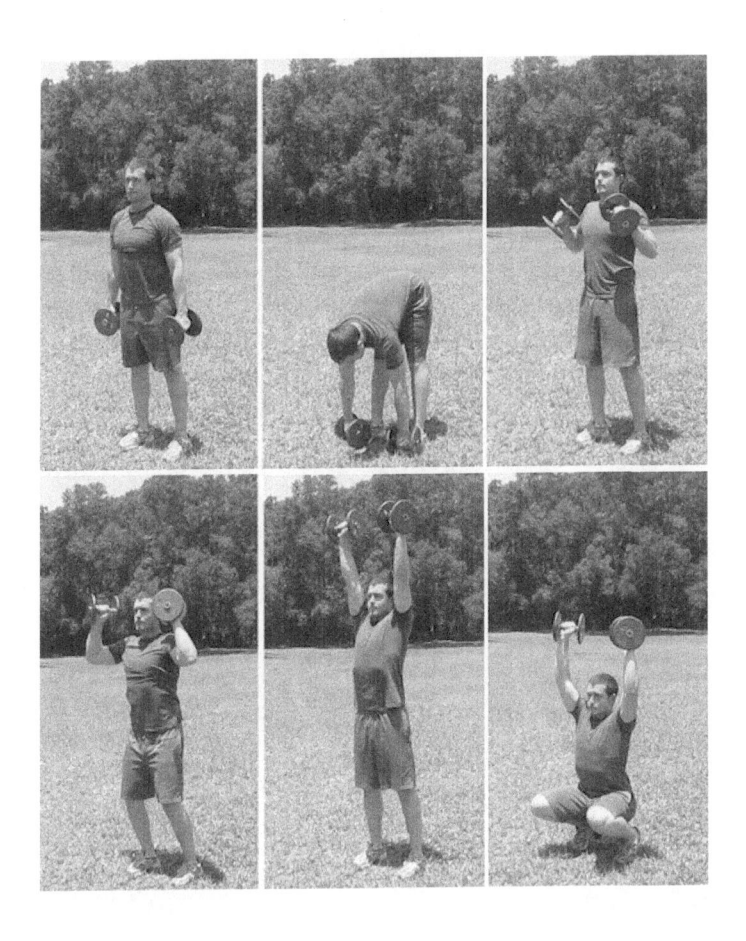

Here's another series of pictures using a barbell, just so you can see how that works:

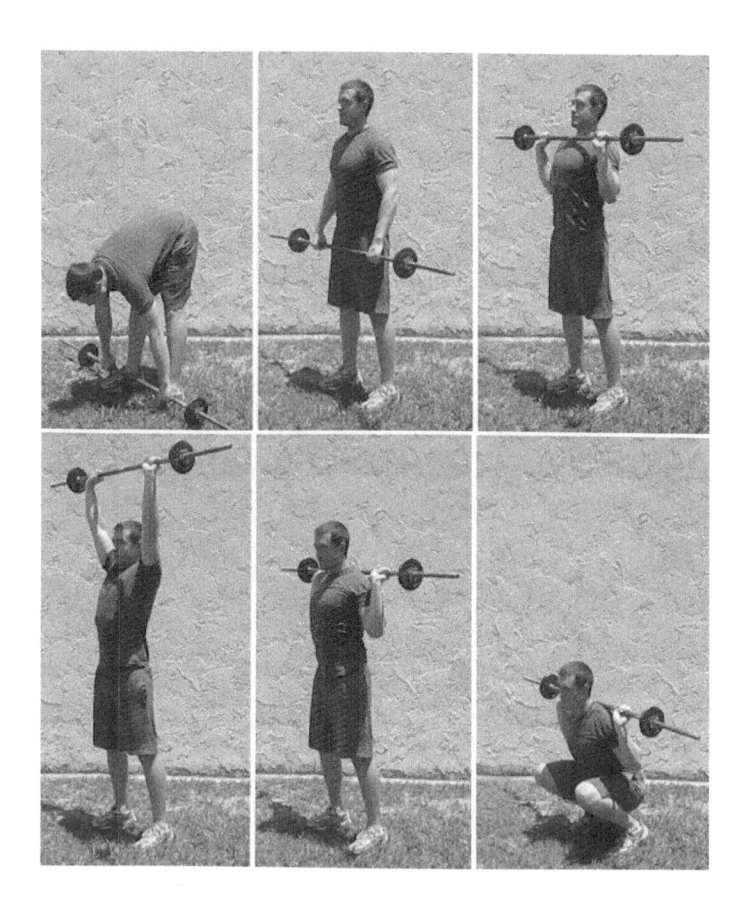

Notice that after the press and before the squat the barbell is lowered behind the neck. Also, the same concept from earlier applies with lowering the weight to your shoulders or keeping it straight above your head during the squat; it's up to you depending on how hard you want it to be.

Choose a weight that you can use for more than a few repetitions. If you're new to exercise, doing 5-10 reps in the beginning will be a challenge. When you're more used to it (or if you're more used to it already), aim for something more in the 12-20 range or more. As you get stronger, increase the repetitions to keep the work challenging. If you get tired of increasing reps, you can get heavier weights to work with, although if you're gauging the repetitions right, you shouldn't need to do that too often.

Depending on your age and experience level you might do this with a total of anywhere from 6-80 pounds, though most people will probably use a total of around 10-40 pounds (that's anywhere from two 5 pound dumbbells to two 20 pound dumbbells, or of course one 10 pound barbell to one 40 pound barbell, just to be clear).

Using weights is up to you. Some people like to add a load to their workouts to make them a little more challenging, although neither method is necessarily better than the other in every case. You can use weights when they're available, and the bodyweight version when they aren't. You can switch back and forth for variety. You can also just forget the whole weights part of this and ignore this chapter if that works better for you.

Using weights obviously makes this motion more challenging, but you will probably do fewer reps with weights than you would without, so the overall work will probably similar, and really, you can get great results using either method, or both. The important thing is that you find the right number of reps of whatever you do so that it's a little bit challenging, and that you make sure you stick with it no matter what.

******

Part 3 concludes the core of this simple workout. If all you want to do is promote your circulation, breathing, and muscle and joint health on a daily basis, that is enough to do it.

Do this sequence with as little rest in between as possible to keep your heartrate up. Some of you may require a short rest if you are not at all used to exercising, and that's fine, although that need should decrease as you do the routine more. If you don't need that, and most of you shouldn't, then just move right from one exercise to the other.

This is not an extremely challenging workout, and its effectiveness depends on the frequency with which you do it. You should do this a minimum of 5 times a week, but really, because it's not very strenuous, there's no reason (unless your doctor gives you one) that you can't do this once every day, which is what I recommend.

In the very beginning you may experience some muscle soreness, especially in your hamstrings, which might make you feel like taking a day off here and there. That's fine, but the soreness should decrease quite a bit as you continue doing the routine, and you should then be able to follow the 5-7 day a week program.

Depending on the exact number of reps, you can have this whole thing done in about two to four minutes.

Everyone has 3 minutes a day, and everyone can benefit from 3 minutes of exercise each day, especially when the alternative is 0 minutes a day, for months or years at a time.

Will this create a quick, dramatic change in your physique by immediately burning fat and building muscle? No. Definitely not. But at 3 minutes a day, it's a feasible workout plan for busy people who might otherwise not exercise at all.

It will help to keep your blood and organs clean, and your joints and muscles useful. If you can take advantage of the convenience of this routine and make it happen on a daily basis (which is the whole point), you'll be much better off a year from now than you would have been if you spent the year being too busy to exercise at all.

If you follow the basic dietary guidelines, you might even see a respectable physical change in a few months to a year. If you decide to incorporate some of the added exercises or tweaks to the schedule that we'll discuss in the coming chapters, you could even see bigger changes more quickly.

PART 4: PUSHUPS/PLANK (OPTIONAL)

Some of you will be looking for more of a challenge than what we've done so far. This part will add a little bit more of an intense upper body and abdominal workout to this routine.

Essentially, we're going to add either one plank or one set of pushups to the routine. Let's look at each of these exercises, and then we'll talk about them. We'll start with the plank.

To do the plank, you will basically hold the up position of a pushup. This exercise will hit your arms, chest, and shoulders, and it will also give you a great abdominal workout—but to make sure you hit your abs, you have to be sure to do the exercise with correct form.

Your body should be straight, and you should be able to flex your abdominal muscles and feel them supporting the weight of your back and your hips. If your hips are too high or too low, you won't have the proper load on your stomach muscles to work them correctly for this exercise.

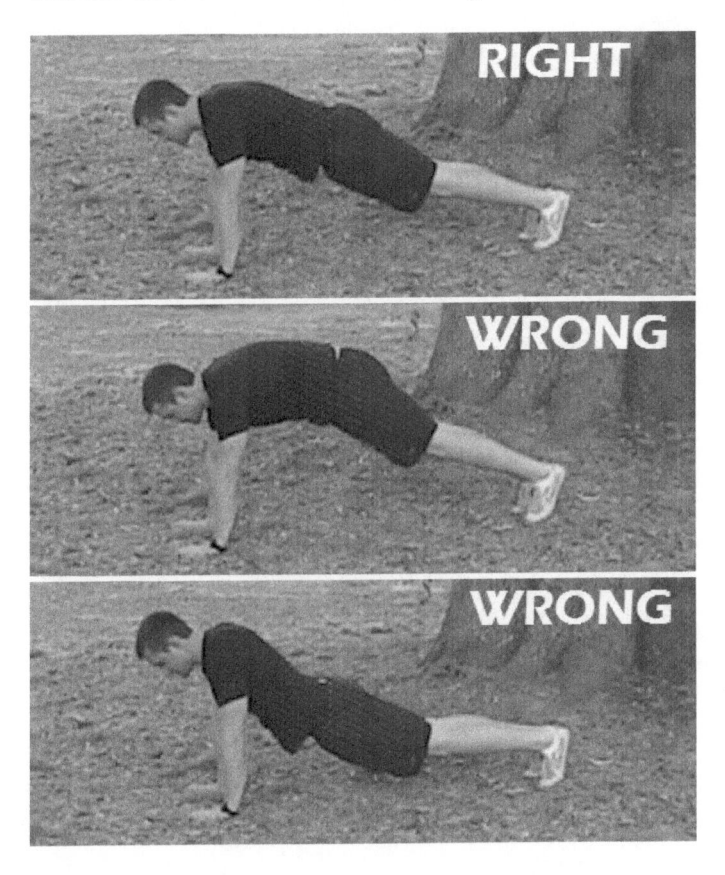

If you aren't familiar with this already, the best thing is to get in as close to the correct position as you can, and flex your abs hard while lifting and dropping your hips just a little bit to feel where the right spot is—you should feel the muscles in your stomach supporting the load of your hips.

Once you get into that position, take deep, slow breaths and hold the position for as long as you comfortably can.

Now we'll look at the other option at this point: the pushup.

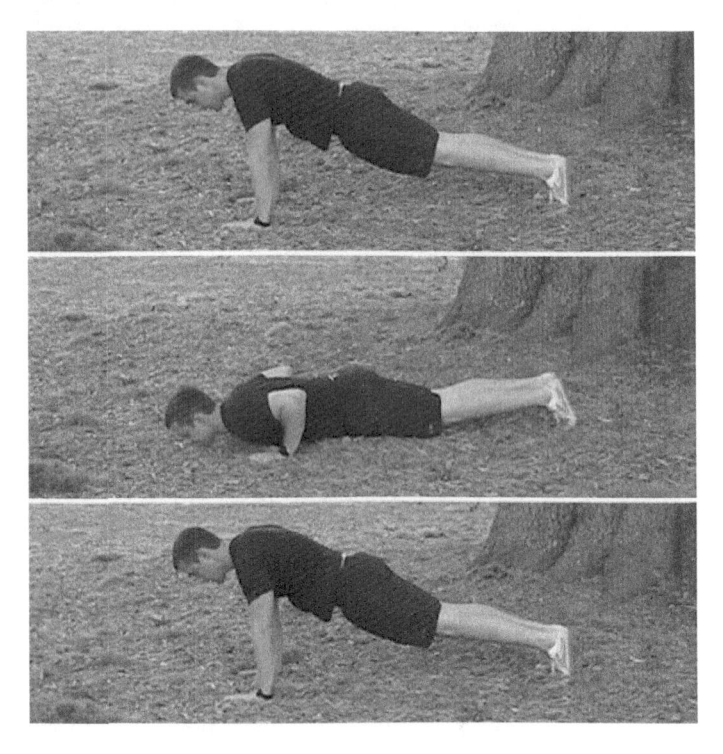

From the plank position we just discussed, simply inhale as you lower yourself until your chest comes just short of touching the floor. Then, exhale and push yourself back up.

If you aren't used to exercise, pushups may be difficult for you, in which case you may want to stick with the plank until you get stronger. Both exercises will work your chest, arms, shoulders, and abs.

If you choose to do the plank, and can't hold it for thirty seconds, just do one plank and hold it for as long as you can. If you can hold it for thirty seconds or longer, you may want to choose a time, probably in the 30-90 second range to keep your workout short and convenient (you can use a stopwatch or just count in your head).

If you choose to do pushups, use the same basic approach to choosing the number of reps as you did for the other exercises. Do enough that it requires some effort, but not so much that you're sweating and gasping for breath. For most people, this will probably fall in the 10-30 pushups range (if you can't do ten pushups yet, just do as many as you can). Of course, if you can, feel free to do 50 or more.

PART 5: CURL PRESS (OPTIONAL)

This is another variation using weights, and like the last weighted exercise, it is extremely optional. If you want a little extra work for your arms and shoulders, this will do it for you. If not, just stick with the regular routine and don't worry about it.

The curl press is great because it's a single exercise that works out all the major muscle groups in your arms, all the way up to your shoulders. It's fairly simple, so just take a look at it on the next page.

As you can see, you will alternate the action on both arms, so you start with one hand already raised in the air.

As you bring that hand down by your side, raise the other arm up so that by the time the first arm is all the way down, the other arm is all the way up.

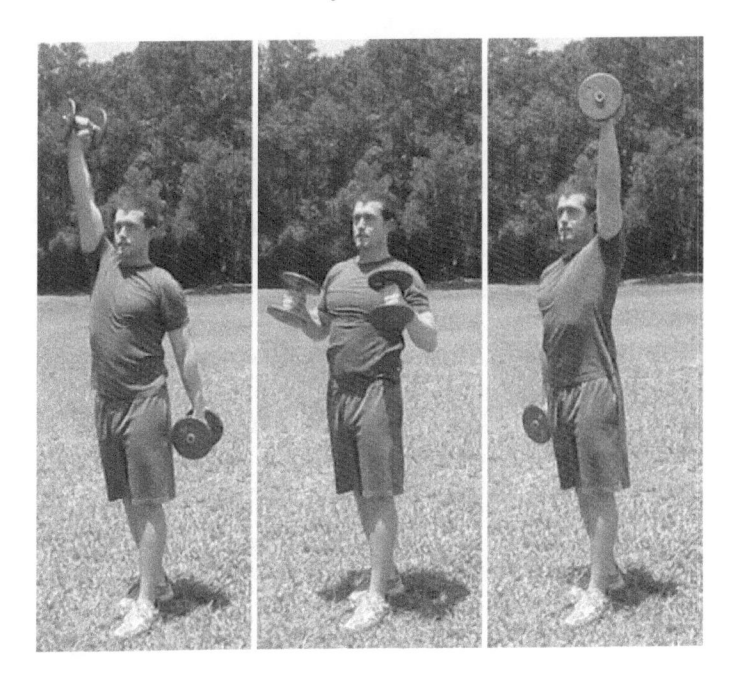

Then, bring the first arm back up and the second arm back down. When you've gotten back to the original position, and each arm has gone up and down once, that's one repetition.

As you can see, whenever one arm is up, the other should be down, and they should be at the same level at about chest height (with one on the way down, and the other one on the way up).

If that's confusing at all, just give it a shot and you'll see what I mean. You can try the movement out right now even if you've got no weights handy, just to get the motion down.

Obviously, this can only be done with two dumbbells, and not with a single barbell, since your hands must move separately from one another.

Be sure to extend your arms all the way up, and all the way back down, and you should stand with one foot slightly forward in front of you, and one foot slighly back for optimal support.

Like the other exercises in this book, this should be executed for one set of a moderate to high number of reps, so use reasonably low weight. Aim for 12-20 reps in the beginning, and if you can't do that without being too sore the next day, drop the weight or drop the reps.

SETS, REPS, AND SCHEDULE

This is maybe the easiest part of this routine, but it's also very important. We'll look at sets first, because it's pretty easy.

Sets

As stated earlier, for each exercise you will do one set. Only doing one set of each exercise means that you do not have to rest between sets, and you do not waste your exercise time waiting around.

Reps

Because you only do one set of each exercise, you need to make it count. That doesn't mean doing the exercise until you collapse, but it does mean pushing yourself a little bit. This is key to the effectiveness of the overall routine, so doing an appropriate number of reps is important.

For beginners, start with low reps. Basically, that means enough reps that you just start to feel comfortable with learning the basic movements in the exercise. Do your reps slowly, and concentrate on each rep as you do it to make sure you get the form right.

Keep things slow and low for the first workout, or the first few workouts, until you feel more comfortable with everything you're doing. Then you want to bump up the reps to a level that's a little bit more challenging.

This gets into sort of the typical range that most people will use. Here's a table with a rough guideline for numbers a lot of people might use.

Jumping Jacks	20-50
Trunk Twists	10-25
Toe Touch Squats	10-25
Pushups (optional)	10-25
Deadlift Press Squats (opt'l)	10-25
Curl Press (optional)	10-25

For some of you, this range will be plenty. All you want to do is get in some daily movement, and these numbers will provide that for you. Every few months you should add a few reps here and there just to keep things interesting, but if you're looking for the basic benefits of this routine—improved circulation, cleaner blood and cells, and so on—this will take care of you.

However, some of you may want something more challenging. We'll discuss a variety of ways to do that, but the most basic way to accomplish that goal is to increase the repetitions more aggressively over time.

This requires you to pay attention, and step things up when your body gets too used to the workout. You can create a schedule—say, add 5 or 10 reps to a given exercise every six or eight weeks—or you can just re-evaluate every so often and adjust accordingly.

For the trunk twists, there's probably not much reason to go higher than about 25 reps in a set. That will accomplish the goal of stretching and activating the muscles in your abs and lower back.

However, for the jumping jacks, toe touch squats, pushups, and so on, you can increase those numbers as much as you can handle them. Although you can benefit from reps in the 10-25 range, you can take any of these exercises up to 50 or 100 reps, or even well beyond that.

It's very easy to be dismissive of simple exercises like toe touches, squats, pushups, and jumping jacks, but remember: some of the fittest people of all time, including Bo Jackson, Herschel Walker, and Jack Lallane, kept in shape by doing hundreds of reps of these types of exercises each day. You don't have to do hundreds to get great results, but don't underestimate the value of increasing the repetitions of these exercises. Not only were these men able to stay in great condition, they also had considerable muscle mass.

I also want to point out that Jack Lallane, although he was in excellent shape as younger man, really started doing his more amazing feats of fitness in his 40s, 50s, and beyond. His example is a great inspiration to anybody who wants to be fit and healthy, regardless of age or prior experience.

If you're motivated, you can get amazing results with high repetitions of these exercises, and since in general adding a repetition means only adding a second or two to the length of your workout, you can still have a very manageable and convenient routine.

One more thing I should note—if you're going to attempt these high reps, be sure to work your way up to them. Don't try for a hundred pushups, or 500 jumping jacks, in your first week of training. Pick something low (as described earlier) to get used to the routine, then increase the reps at a rate that is comfortable over the next few weeks and months. There's no rush to get to the high reps —the important thing is just to get in that daily work, keep your training a little bit challenging, and don't get into anything you aren't ready for.

Schedule

Now that we've looked at your sets and reps, we'll talk about the schedule. By now, you've probably picked up on the fact that this is intended to be a daily workout routine. Because you'll be doing light exercise, you need to do it every day for it to be effective, or at least a minimum of 5 days a week (whichever five days you like).

In the very beginning, if you aren't used to exercise at all (or if you aren't used to these exercises), you may have some soreness and you might want to wait a day or two between workouts. In particular, you might be surprised at the soreness in your hamstrings from the toe touch motion.

Again, that's perfectly fine and normal, and at first you might want to do the routine every other day or so, or only do the toe touch squats every third day, or something like that.

However, once you are in full swing, there's nothing to stop you from doing this routine every day, and in fact that's kind of the point of this book. While it's true that heavier, more traditional routines require a day (or more) of rest between similar workouts, this light exercise routine is designed to be effective when done 5-7 times a week.

We'll discuss the importance and necessity of rest in more detail in the next chapter, but for now just think of this as basically a daily routine.

******

That was a pretty in-depth explanation, so I'll sum it up for you in two sentences: Do one set of each exercise, in the order described, every day. Do enough repetitions that the exercise is challenging, but not so many that it extremely difficult.

Now let's get a little deeper understanding of the importance of rest, and how it relates to this routine.

REST

I know there will be some people who cry foul when I talk about doing the same exercise routine each day, so I wanted to include this short chapter on rest to make sure we're all on the same page.

In a traditional exercise routine, you train your muscles more heavily. They break down, and they need some time to rest and get repaired before they can do that hard work again. If they don't get the rest they need, you can overtrain your muscles and cause injury or other problems.

However, not every exercise routine hits this threshold that requires at least a day of repair. Let's consider an example to illustrate this point. Obviously, most people walk around during the day. Walking around is physical exercise, but you don't need to take the next day off from walking to recover, do you? Walking around for a day is just not intense enough to require taking the next day off. This routine, although more intense than just an ordinary walk, should be the same way.

Your body can handle walking around one day, and doing more walking the next. Similarly, your body can handle doing a set of jumping jacks one day, and doing another set the next day, and the next day. If you tried to break a world record by doing thousands of jumping jacks in a row, you would need at least a few days rest after that—but that's not what we're doing here.

The key here is to monitor your own body, and that's important if you're doing this exercise routine or any other.

There are two key situations to look out for where you might need a little bit of rest, and both involve paying attention to soreness in your body.

You might notice soreness in the beginning in certain muscles if you aren't used to using them. If you notice that soreness, feel free to wait a day or two (or more) until the soreness is mostly gone—it's not necessary for it to be 100 percent gone, but you can wait until you feel comfortable doing more exercise. As you do more of these workouts your muscles should get accustomed to the work and you should feel less soreness, which should allow you to get on the 5-7 times a week track with no trouble.

The other situation where you might need more rest is if your goal is to "push yourself" with this routine (using some of the variations we've already discussed, or some we will discuss in the next chapter). If you want to try much higher reps, or if you're trying several of the more advanced options, then you may find yourself to be pretty sore. The remedy is the same—give yourself a day or two of added rest until the soreness decreases.

However, if you want to stick to this routine, you should not regularly do exercise that is so strenuous that it requires multiple days of rest. If you are unable to do this routine for at least four days out of the week, you should decrease your number of repetitions (or otherwise make the routine easier) until you can get back in the 5-7 days a week range, or you should find a different program to follow.

You can certainly have success by working out 3 or 4 times a week, but if you decide to do that you're really getting away from the purpose and structure of this workout plan; the advice you find here will start to be less relevant, and you should learn a different kind of routine.

For the absolute best results, you want to try to find that sweet spot where you're doing enough repetitions that you're getting in some work, but not quite so many that you have any significant soreness the next day. That way you're progressing a little bit all the time, which can have an enormous impact in the long run.

In order to find that sweet spot, you have to experiment to find the right numbers. In other words, you need to pay attention to the physical results of what you're doing on a daily basis.

If you think you might not be getting enough work, increase your numbers a little bit each day. When you start to feel that slight soreness the next day, that will tell you that you're hovering right around the sweet spot; if the soreness is anything more than slight, back off on the number of reps a little bit. If you start to feel like you're not working hard enough a few weeks later, bump up those numbers a little bit again.

Easy Exercises

As long as you're near that sweet spot, a simple night's rest should be plenty to get you in shape to do your short workout the next day, and if you find that you need to take a day or two off during the week (doesn't matter which days), that's fine as long as you follow the guidelines in this chapter and in the rest of this book.

CHALLENGE YOURSELF

In this chapter, you will learn about a few simple variations you can try to mix in to create a greater physical challenge for yourself with this workout.

Now, bear in mind that the ultimate goal with all of this is just to promote daily exercise, so you don't want to take yourself out of commission with anything too intense. However, adding a little bit of an extra challenge once or twice a week will get you even better results, and if you do get a little bit sore, you can always take off a day or two to get back on track, as previously discussed.

Also, if you start mixing in these challenges with more frequency, you may find that you can do them on a daily (or almost daily) basis without taxing yourself too much—in other words, you'll get stronger and healthier enough that what used to be a difficult challenge can become your daily routine!

Easy Exercises

The simplest way to challenge yourself has already been discussed—add repetitions over time as you get to be in better condition.

Another way we've already discussed is to add the plank or pushup element into your workout. If you aren't doing that now, try to add it in once or twice a week, and you may find that you can do it without trouble as part of your normal routine.

One convenient way to get more of the exercise in is just to find another time to do the whole routine at a different point in the day. If you're used to doing it in the morning right after you wake up, then do it again before dinner, or before bed. The rest between workouts during the day should mean you'll have no trouble doing another round.

Start off by doing this once or twice a week, but over time you might decide to do it three or four times a week, or even every day.

You can also do the whole routine straight through twice, or do the routine once and just double the reps (doing the whole routine through twice will be slightly easier because you'll get a little rest between the two sets of each movement).

This may be a little less convenient because you might start to sweat, which could be a pain at the office or while getting ready in the morning. It will obviously take twice as long; it's probably easier to find two four minute periods during the day when you can exercise than it is to find one eight minute period. So, this one might be better to try on the weekend or when you have a little more time than normal.

You can also pick an exercise each day to add a few reps to, just for that day. If you normally do 40 jumping jacks, try 75 one day. The next day go back to 40 jumping jacks, but try 15 pushups instead of 10. The next day go back to 40 jumping jacks and 10 pushups, but try 25 toe touch squats instead of 15, and so on. That way you're rotating which exercise is more challenging each day, so you're getting a better workout without ever wearing down your whole body so much that you delay recovery.

You could take that same concept but do a weekly rotation: spend a week doing higher numbers on jumping jacks, then drop them to normal the next week and up your numbers on the toe touch squats, and so on.

As you can see, the ideas are potentially endless, but they come down to two basic elements—find some way to increase the work you're doing, and do it with some kind of logic or structure, so that it's easy to keep doing it.

DON'T UNDERVALUE THIS

This workout routine is simple, but I am not exaggerating when I say it could change your life.

Do you know what the difference is between people who stay in pretty good (or even great) shape, and people who are always dealing with high weight and low energy? There is no secret exercise or food. In almost every situation, the difference is that the people in good shape have found something they can stick to.

If you bought this book, then on some level you must still be looking for that program you can stick to. Well, this is about as simple as it gets, without being too easy or too limited. If this is the program that takes you from being too busy to work out to being able to work out on a daily basis, then that simple change is beyond huge.

Maybe it's a jumping-off point that allows you to pursue grander goals of fitness. Or, maybe this is exactly what you need just how it is, and you stick with it indefinitely. Either way, the key to everything is consistent effort.

Let's think about what would have happened if you found this book a year ago, and applied it then. Let's take a fairly conservative guess and imagine that you would have averaged 25 jumping jacks, 10 trunk twists, 15 toe touch squats, and just 5 pushups a day for the last year. Here's what you would have under your belt now:

Jumping Jacks	9,125
Trunk Twists	3,650
Toe Touch Squats	5,475
Pushups	1,825

Using this simple routine, and without going to a gym (or otherwise going out of your way at all), in just a few minutes a day you would be more than 9,000 jumping jacks, more than 3,600 trunk twists, almost 5,500 toe touches and squats, and nearly 2,000 pushups better off than you are right now, as you read this.

That's more than 20,000 repetitions of bodyweight exercise in a year by just taking a few minutes out of each day—and most of you could probably beat those numbers by 50-100% or more if you pushed it just a tiny bit.

Take a minute to think about how much better your body would look and feel if you had done that. Think about the strength and energy you would have each day—the strength and energy you would have right now.

Seriously. Stop and think about it for a minute.

Easy Exercises

This routine is so powerful not because it contains some secret formula, but because it is simple and complete and anybody can use it. So please, use it! Start today so that a year from now you can see and feel the results of those 20,000+ repetitions.

Busy people start to be out of shape when days and weeks of no exercise turn into months and years of no exercise. Avoid this dangerous trap, stay strong and healthy, and put this simple program to work.

EASY EXERCISE AS A SUPPLEMENT

If you're a little more experienced when it comes to fitness, there's another way you can use this program—in fact, it's the way I often use it.

You can use this program to supplement a broader exercise routine. For example, if you already make it to the gym 3 times a week for a longer workout, you can still add in this program 5-7 days a week to get in even better shape without taking much extra time out of your day.

Then, if you're extra busy, or away from home, or otherwise unable to maintain your normal gym-going schedule, you can easily keep up this short daily exercise routine so you don't slip into the dangerous habit of putting off exercise until you've got less 'stuff' going on.

Conversely, if you've never been one for a lot of exercise, starting with this routine might lead you to longer, more involved workouts. Even as you start to add those into your routine, you can still stick to what we've talked about in this book as a solid and reliable foundation for regular exercise.

Whether this is the only exercise you do, or it's just part of the exercise you do, it's a routine that is dependable, convenient, and valuable—so find a way to incorporate it into whatever fitness regimen you follow.

BASIC DIET

Okay, this book teaches you a stripped-down, simple, easy-to-apply bodyweight (or limited weight) exercise routine, so let's take a look at a stripped-down, simple, easy-to-use approach to your diet.

The world of nutrition is tough to navigate. Everybody has a different opinion about what works, and it seems like everybody's opinion changes every month or so. However, you need to understand whats going to help you shed excess weight and support lean muscle if you want the best results from this routine.

There are fads and trends that come and go constantly, so we'll talk about three simple, core ideas that you can always come back to any time you're feeling confused. It's hard to pick the best one, so we'll say they're all equally important.

1) Drink Water

That should maybe be "Drink Water Instead Of Whatever Else You're Drinking." Your body desperately needs water. That means just regular water, not flavored water, not soda that contains carbonated water, just water.

Every day inside your body there are thousands, maybe tens or hundreds of thousands of tiny processes that must happen to keep you alive and healthy. Most of them require water, and if you don't drink it, you're going to be in trouble.

Also, if you're not drinking water, you might be drinking soda (or worse, diet soda), or sweet tea, or processed fruit juices, or who knows what else. For the most part, drinking anything but water means sucking down processed sugar, or artificial sweeteners, or food additives, or more realistically a combination of the three.

Drink plenty of water each day. Outside of fruits or vegetables you're going to juice yourself, or organic cow's milk, I wouldn't drink much else. You'll avoid plenty of unwanted sugar and additives, and you'll give your body the water it needs to perform at a peak level.

2) Eat Fruit

Fresh fruit is the best fuel you can give your body. It's very important that when I say fresh fruit, you understand that I'm talking about actual fresh unprocessed fruit from the produce section, or from a produce market. We are not talking about fruit slices packed in syrup, or fruit leather, or anything except a piece of fruit that's in the same condition it was in when it came off of the tree, or the vine, or the bush it was grown on.

As important as fresh fruit is, it's amazing that many people consume almost none on a regular basis. Strive to eat at least some fresh fruit—any kind you like—with every meal. It's easy for your body to digest, and it's loaded with healthy carbohydrates and all kinds of vitamins and minerals that are hard to get elsewhere.

You need fruit. Eat it every day.

3) Avoid Processed Foods

You've heard this before, I'm sure, but it might be difficult for you to appreciate how very important it is. Start reading the labels on foods, and as an easy rule of thumb, go with the foods that have the fewest number of ingredients. When you see a food that has dozens of ingredients, including artifical colors and flavors, look for an alternative or forget it altogether.

The best foods have one ingredient—an apple, or a piece of fish, for example. You can see plainly what they are, and there's nothing to worry about hiding under the surface. Try to make sures your diet consists of as many of these types of foods as possible.

******

So those are pretty simple rules: drink water, eat fruit, avoid processed stuff. Just like the exercise routine, they are simple but powerful, and you can see great rewards if you stick with them.

Oh, and be sure you're getting protein in your diet—with these exercises your body will be building a little muscle now, so (especially if you're not used to regular exercise) you'll need to be sure you're eating protein from whichever combination of meat, fish, nuts, beans, eggs, and dairy you prefer.

If you want a more complete explanation of the best things to eat—and not to eat—you might want to pick up a copy of my book on the subject, The Natural Diet. It's a focused and logical approach to human nutrition, and I think you'll find it makes a lot more sense than most of what's out there.

Even if you don't read that book, though, these three tips are plenty to get you on the right path, so start using them.

GENERAL TIPS

As I've said a few times, the key to this (or any) workout routine is sticking with it. Because it's short and doesn't require any equipment, this is an easy one to stick to, but one thing that can help is picking a certain time each day that you always do your exercises.

For a lot of people, the best time is in the morning before school or work. It might also be when you get home, or right before dinner, or before you go to bed. If you've worked your way up to it, you might even pick two of those times to do it.

Whatever it is, though, pick it and stick to it. Soon it will be automatic, like putting on your socks or brushing your teeth. It will become something you just do, and the results will come, slow and steady and lasting.

Fresh air and exercise are powerful. They can even be powerful in small quantities, especially compared to not getting them at all.

Easy Exercises

Adding little things, like a walk outside, can make a difference. Grab your dog or your significant other or your pet rock or whatever and just get outside a few times a week, even for 20 minutes. You could join a recreational sports league, start swimming, almost anything you do regularly makes a difference, and (if possible) finding someone who will do it with you helps a lot too.

Your body is made to move, and movement will keep you healthy. Keep moving, and keep eating right, and you'll be glad you did.

CONCLUSION

Well, that's it. You now know everything you need to know to follow a simple, effective workout routine in just a few minutes a day.

As with any effective workout routine, the only secret is sticking to it. Since you're finishing the book right now, I'd recommend that you get up after the end of this chapter and do your very first workout from this book.

If you took the time to read this book, I have to assume on some level it's because you weren't happy with your current knowledge of exercise, and you didn't feel like you had a worthwhile routine that you could fit into your day. Now you know the routine, you know enough about what you should be eating and not eating, and the only thing left to do is get started.

So do it! Put down this book and get started right now.

ABOUT THE AUTHOR

Patrick Barrett has been interested in exercise ever since he started to lift weights with his dad and older brothers as a kid. He participated in a half-dozen organized sports (most notably inline hockey and high school wrestling) until a neck injury during a wrestling match in his junior year prevented him from playing further in any contact sports.

After the injury, he developed an interest in pursuing strength and balance, particularly through bodyweight and self-taught gymnastic-type exercises.

Patrick has always loved both cooking and eating food. Unsatisfied with the confusing and often contradictory nutritional advice offered by mainstream sources, Patrick searched for another way to understand human nutrition that was logical, consistent, and effective. His books on food and nutrition reflect this 'cleaner,' more intuitive and useful understanding of food and how it impacts our health.

Patrick hopes that his books will save his audience time and aggravation by finally offering practical ways to achieve their nutrition and fitness goals.

OTHER BOOKS BY PATRICK BARRETT

Natural Exercise: *Basic Bodyweight Training and Calisthenics for Strength and Weight-Loss*

Advanced Bodyweight Exercises: *An Intense Full Body Workout In A Home Or Gym*

The Natural Diet: *Simple Nutritional Advice For Optimal Health In The Modern World*

How To Do A Handstand: *From the Basic Exercises To The Free Standing Handstand Pushup*

Best Ab Exercises: *Abdominal Workout Routine For Core Strength And A Flat Stomach*

Hand And Forearm Exercises: *Grip Strength Workout And Training Routine*

One Arm Pull Up: *Bodyweight Training And Exercise Program For One Arm Pull Ups And Chin Ups*

CPSIA information can be obtained at www.ICGtesting.com
Printed in the USA
LVOW011831180613

339165LV00025B/885/P

9 781478 200277